DYSPHAGIA COOKBOOK FOR SENIORS

Savoring Soft Delights, Nourishing Recipes for Seniors with Dysphagia"

Magdalene Charles

DYSPHAGIA
COOKBOOK
FOR SENIORS

Savoring Soft Delights
Nourishing Recipes
for Seniors with
Dysphagia"

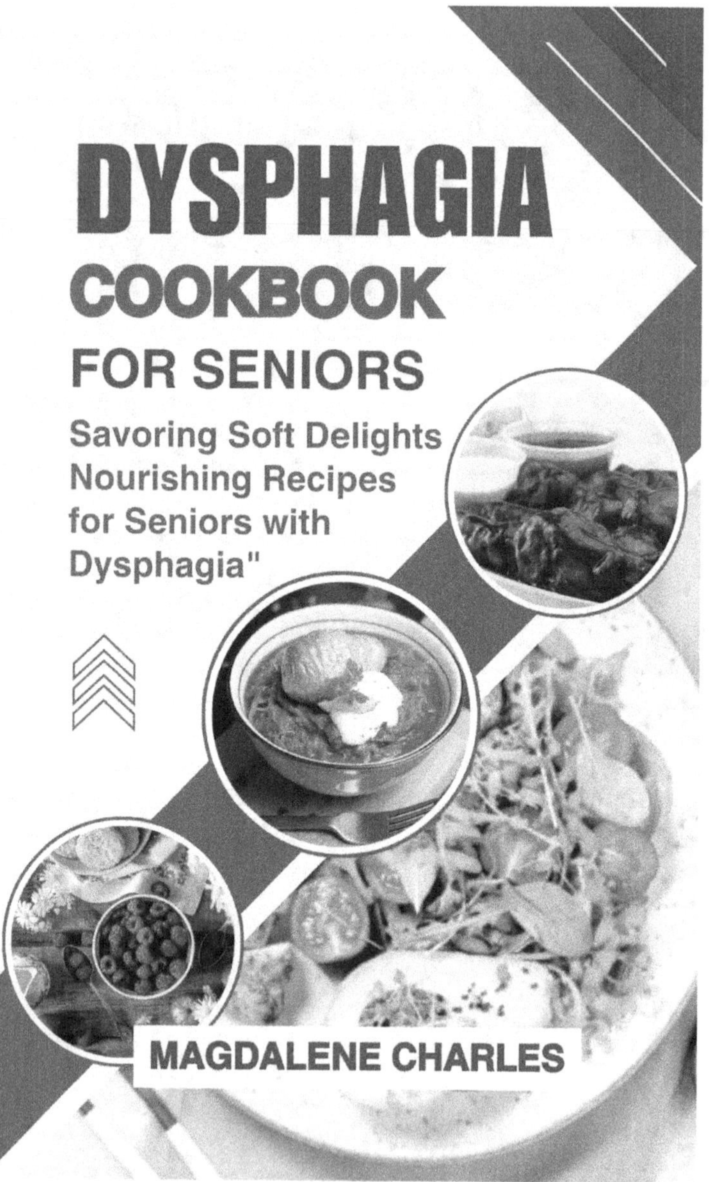

MAGDALENE CHARLES

TABLE OF CONTENT

OVERVIEW

Welcome to "Savoring Soft Delights: Nourishing Recipes for Seniors with Dysphagia." This cookbook is crafted with care and culinary expertise to meet the unique needs of seniors facing the challenges of dysphagia, a condition that affects swallowing. We understand that maintaining a healthy and enjoyable diet is essential for overall well-being, and this collection of recipes aims to make the dining experience not only nourishing but also delightful.

Dysphagia, a condition commonly associated with aging, can make eating a daunting task, impacting both the physical and emotional aspects of an individual's life. Swallowing difficulties may arise due to various factors such as neurological disorders, muscle weakness, or other medical conditions. Recognizing the importance of adapting to these challenges, "Savoring Soft Delights" provides a selection of recipes that focus on textures and flavors suitable for those with dysphagia, ensuring that meals remain a source of joy and sustenance.

In this introductory section, we will explore the significance of understanding dysphagia, the vital role of nutrition in the lives of seniors, and the thoughtful approach taken to tailor each recipe for optimal swallowing comfort. Whether you are a caregiver seeking nutritious and easy-to-swallow options for your loved one or an individual navigating dysphagia, this cookbook is designed to empower you with a diverse range of delectable choices that prioritize both health and taste.

As we embark on this culinary journey together, let "Savoring Soft Delights" be your guide to creating meals that not only nourish the body but also celebrate the pleasure of eating. With a focus on soft textures, rich flavors, and nutritional value, these recipes aim to transform mealtimes into moments of comfort, satisfaction, and, above all, enjoyment.

May this cookbook bring warmth to your kitchen, joy to your dining table, and, most importantly, a renewed sense of culinary delight for seniors with dysphagia.

CHAPTER 1

SMOOTH STARTERS

Creamy Vegetable Soup

Ingredients:

- 1 cup carrots, peeled and diced
- 1 cup potatoes, peeled and chopped
- 1 cup zucchini, sliced
- 1/2 cup celery, finely chopped
- 1/2 cup onion, finely diced
- 2 cloves garlic, minced
- 4 cups low-sodium vegetable broth
- 1 cup low-fat milk or non-dairy milk alternative
- 2 tablespoons unsalted butter or olive oil
- Salt and pepper to taste
- Fresh herbs for garnish (such as parsley or chives)

Instructions:

- Sauté Aromatics: Melt butter or warm up olive oil in a big saucepan over medium heat. Add the minced garlic and diced onions, and cook until aromatic and transparent.

- Add Vegetables: Add celery, carrots, potatoes, and zucchini to the saucepan. Cook the vegetables for five to seven minutes, stirring now and then.

- Pour Broth: Make sure the vegetables are covered with the low-sodium vegetable broth as you pour it in. After bringing the mixture to a mild boil, lower the heat so that it simmers. Let the veggies simmer until they are soft.

- Blend to Smooth Consistency: Gently blend the soup with an immersion blender until it's smooth. Alternatively, move the soup in batches to make sure it's not too hot to a blender and process until the consistency is creamy.

- Add Milk: Slowly pour in the nondairy milk or low-fat milk, stirring to fully incorporate it into the soup. To taste, add salt and pepper for seasoning.

- Pour the creamy vegetable soup into dishes and garnish with parsley. Add some fresh herbs, such chives or parsley, as a garnish for a taste and visual boost.

Silky Butternut Squash Bisque

Ingredients:

- 1 medium-sized butternut squash, peeled, seeded, and diced
- 1 onion, chopped
- 2 carrots, peeled and sliced

- 2 apples, peeled, cored, and chopped
- 4 cups low-sodium chicken or vegetable broth
- 1 cup low-fat coconut milk or regular milk
- 2 tablespoons olive oil
- 1 teaspoon ground ginger
- 1/2 teaspoon ground nutmeg
- Salt and pepper to taste
- Roasted pumpkin seeds for garnish (optional)

Instructions:

- Prepare the vegetables by heating the olive oil in a large pot over medium heat. Add the diced apples, carrots, and onions. Vegetables should be sautéed until tender and aromatic.

- Add Butternut Squash: Stir the chopped butternut squash into the sautéed mixture after adding it to the pot.

- Season and Simmer: Dust the vegetables with nutmeg and ground ginger. To taste, add salt and pepper for seasoning. Make sure the veggies are submerged in the low-sodium broth before adding more. After bringing the mixture to a low boil, lower the heat so that it simmers. Simmer the mixture until the butternut squash is soft.

- Blend to Silky Smoothness: Blend the ingredients in batches in a blender or with an immersion blender until it reaches a silky smooth consistency. Take care not to combine hot liquids; if needed, let the soup cool somewhat.

- Add Coconut Milk: To give the bisque a hint of smoothness, stir in either standard or low-fat coconut milk. If necessary, adjust the seasoning.

- Pour the Silky Butternut Squash Bisque into dishes and garnish with parsley. To enhance the flavor and visual appeal, scatter roasted pumpkin seeds over the dish.

Pureed Spinach and Potato Delight

Ingredients:

- 2 cups fresh spinach, washed and chopped
- 2 large potatoes, peeled and diced
- 1 onion, finely chopped
- 2 cloves garlic, minced
- 3 cups low-sodium vegetable or chicken broth
- 1 cup low-fat milk or non-dairy milk alternative
- 2 tablespoons olive oil
- Salt and pepper to taste

- Nutmeg for a hint of warmth (optional)
- Fresh chives for garnish

Instructions:

- Sauté Aromatics: Place a big saucepan over medium heat with olive oil. Add the minced garlic and chopped onions, and sauté until fragrant and translucent.

- Add the potatoes: Add the chopped potatoes to the saucepan and toss to coat them with the browned mixture.

- Pour in Broth: Fill the pot with low-sodium chicken or vegetable broth, making sure the potatoes are covered. After bringing the mixture to a boil, lower the heat so that it simmers. Cook the potatoes until they are quite soft.

- Add the spinach and let it wilt into the mixture by tossing it in. Cook the spinach for a further three to five minutes, or until it is soft.

- Blend to Puree: Puree the contents in batches in a blender or with an immersion blender until a creamy consistency is reached.

- Add Milk: To ensure a creamy consistency, whisk in the non dairy or low-fat milk. To taste, add salt and pepper for seasoning. If you want an additional layer of warmth, add a pinch of nutmeg.

- Pour the Pureed Spinach and Potato Delight into dishes for serving and garnishing. Add some fresh chives as a garnish for some color and extra freshness.

Avocado and Yogurt Smoothie

Ingredients:

- 1 ripe avocado, peeled and pitted
- 1 cup plain Greek yogurt or a non-dairy alternative
- 1 banana, peeled
- 1 cup almond milk or any preferred milk
- 1 tablespoon honey or maple syrup (optional for sweetness)
- Ice cubes for a chilled consistency

Instructions:

- To prepare the avocado, scoop out the flesh and transfer it to a blender.

- Add Yogurt and Banana: Start with the peeled banana and then add plain Greek yogurt or a non dairy substitute.

- Pour in Milk: For a smooth consistency, add your favorite milk or almond milk to the blender.

- Sweeten (Optional): For a little sweetness, add some honey or maple syrup. To suit your tastes, adjust the sweetness.

- Blend to Perfection: Process the ingredients in a blender until a silky, smooth texture is reached. If needed, incorporate ice cubes to make a cool and revitalizing smoothie.

- Present and Savor: Transfer the Avocado and Yogurt Smoothie into a glass and relish its rich, velvety flavor.

This smoothie is a nutritional powerhouse that also satisfies the textural requirements of people who have dysphagia. Yogurt provides a creamy richness and healthful bacteria, while avocado offers a dose of heart-healthy fats and a velvety texture. The natural sweetness and creamy texture of the banana add to the pleasant, satiating, and healthy beverage.

The Avocado and Yogurt Smoothie perfectly captures the spirit of "Savoring Soft Delights," whether it is consumed as a midday snack, morning booster, or addition to a well-balanced meal plan. It turns the idea of a straightforward smoothie into a sensory experience, demonstrating that pleasure and health can coexist in one delicious drink especially when it comes to recipes that are friendly to dysphagia.

CHAPTER 2

APPETIZING APPETIZERS

Mashed Avocado Bruschetta

Ingredients:

- 1 ripe avocado, peeled and pitted
- 1 tablespoon fresh lemon juice
- 1 clove garlic, minced
- Salt and pepper to taste
- 1 tablespoon extra-virgin olive oil
- 1 loaf of soft French bread or a dysphagia-friendly bread alternative
- Fresh basil leaves for garnish (optional)
- Cherry tomatoes, halved, for topping (optional)

Instructions:

- To make Mashed Avocado, mash the ripe avocado with a fork in a bowl. Add the minced garlic, lemon juice, salt, and pepper. Blend until well mixed, resulting in a creamy and aromatic avocado mash.

- Cut the soft French bread or a substitute that is dysphagia-friendly into slices and toast it. Toast the pieces until they become golden brown and become crisp, but not crunchy.

- Spread Avocado Mash: To create a smooth, creamy layer, liberally spread the mashed avocado mixture over each slice of toast.

- Drizzle with Olive Oil: To add a hint of richness and depth to the dish, drizzle extra-virgin olive oil over the mashed avocado.

- Garnish (Optional): Add some fresh basil leaves or cut cherry tomatoes to the Mashed Avocado Bruschetta for a pop of color and freshness.

- To serve and savor, place the bruschetta on a platter and enjoy the lovely blend of toasted bread, creamy avocado, and garlicky bliss.

Whipped Hummus with Soft Pita

Ingredients:

For Whipped Hummus:

- 1 can (15 ounces) chickpeas, drained and rinsed
- 1/4 cup tahini
- 2 cloves garlic, minced
- 3 tablespoons extra-virgin olive oil
- 2 tablespoons fresh lemon juice
- 1/2 teaspoon ground cumin
- Salt and pepper to taste
- Water (as needed for consistency)

For Soft Pita:

- Soft, dysphagia-friendly pita bread

Instructions:

For Whipped Hummus:

- To prepare the chickpeas, place them in a food processor together with the tahini, minced garlic, fresh lemon juice, extra-virgin olive oil, ground cumin, salt, and pepper.
- Blend to Smooth Consistency: Mix the ingredients in a processor until a creamy, smooth consistency is reached. Water can be added gradually to the hummus to get the desired texture if it's too thick.
- Taste the hummus and make any required adjustments to the spices. To taste, adjust with extra salt, pepper, or lemon juice.

Regarding Soft Pita:

- Warm Pita Bread: Use a microwave or oven to gently reheat the malleable, soft pita bread that is suitable for those with dysphagia.
- Cut into Bite-Sized Pieces: To make eating the warmed pita bread easier, cut it into bite-sized pieces.

To Serve:

- Present Whipped Hummus: To make a smooth and enticing base, spoon the whipped hummus onto a serving dish.
- Arrange Soft Pita: Place the small, bite-sized soft pita pieces around the whipped hummus so that they are ready to be dipped and enjoyed.
- Garnish (Optional): Add a pinch of ground cumin and a drizzle of extra-virgin olive oil to the whipped hummus for a visual pop.

- **Serve and Enjoy:** Savor the comfortable softness of pita bread and the creamy richness of hummus as you sink your teeth into this delicious combination of whipped hummus and soft pita.

Pimento Cheese Spread on Soft Crackers

Ingredients:

For Pimento Cheese Spread:

- 1 cup shredded sharp cheddar cheese
- 1/2 cup mayonnaise
- 1/4 cup diced pimentos, drained
- 1 tablespoon finely grated onion
- 1 teaspoon Dijon mustard
- 1/2 teaspoon Worcestershire sauce
- Salt and pepper to taste

For Soft Crackers:

- Soft, dysphagia-friendly crackers

Instructions:

For Pimento Cheese Spread:

- Ingredients: Combine mayonnaise, diced pimentos, finely grated onion, Dijon mustard, Worcestershire sauce, shredded sharp cheddar cheese, salt, and pepper in a mixing dish.

- Mix to Creamy Consistency: Use a whisk to combine the ingredients and work them into a smooth, creamy mixture. To suit your tastes, adjust the seasoning.

Regarding Soft Crackers:

- Pick Crackers That Are Dysphagia-Friendly: Select easy-to-eat, soft crackers that are mild on the palate for people with dysphagia.

- Arrange Crackers: Arrange the delicate crackers in a dish or plate, prepared to be topped with the rich spread of pimento cheese.

To Serve:

- Spread Pimento Cheese: To make a tasty and savory topping, liberally spread the pimento cheese mixture onto each soft cracker using a butter knife or spoon.

- Garnish (Optional): Add some finely chopped chives or paprika to the Pimento Cheese Spread for an additional visual pop.

- Serve and Enjoy: Savor the rich, tangy flavors of the cheese spread and the soft, mild crunch of the crackers as you tuck into this delicious combination of Pimento Cheese Spread on Soft Crackers.

Zucchini and Goat Cheese Bites

Ingredients:

- 2 medium-sized zucchinis, finely grated
- 4 ounces goat cheese, softened
- 2 tablespoons finely chopped fresh herbs (such as basil, chives, or parsley)
- 1 clove garlic, minced
- 1 tablespoon extra-virgin olive oil
- Salt and pepper to taste
- Dysphagia-friendly bread or crackers for serving (optional)

Instructions:

- Get the zucchini ready:Grate the zucchini finely, then transfer them to a fresh kitchen towel. Remove as much moisture as possible from the shredded zucchini.
- Mix the ingredients together:Grated zucchini, softened goat cheese,

minced garlic, finely chopped fresh herbs, extra-virgin olive oil, salt, and pepper should all be combined in a mixing dish.

- Blend to Create a Blend:Mixing the ingredients together will ensure that the goat cheese is uniformly dispersed throughout the well-combined batter.
- Form into Bits:Form the mixture into bite-sized quantities using a spoon or your hands to form tiny, round patties or bites.
- Relax (Optional):You can refrigerate the goat cheese and zucchini bites for around half an hour to give them a firmer texture.
- Serve:Place the Goat Cheese and Zucchini Bites in a serving tray. They can be eaten on their own or with crackers or toast that is suitable for dysphagia.

- Optional garnish:Add a drizzle of olive oil or more fresh herbs as a decorative touch to the bites.
- Present and Savor: Savor the subtle fusion of mild zucchini and the creamy, tangy notes of goat cheese as you dive into the culinary delight that is zucchini and goat cheese bites.

This adaption is dysphagia-friendly and offers a delicious combination of flavors and textures. The richness of goat cheese and the fragrant herbs combine with the soft zucchini to create a flavorful and easily ingested sensory experience. These morsels capture the spirit of "Savoring Soft Delights," making them a great appetizer or a delightful snack that seniors with special dietary needs can enjoy and easily consume.

CHAPTER 3

TENDER PROTEINS

Slow-Cooked Shredded Chicken

Ingredients:

- 2 pounds boneless, skinless chicken breasts or thighs
- 1 onion, finely chopped
- 2 cloves garlic, minced
- 1 cup low-sodium chicken broth
- 1 teaspoon dried thyme
- 1 teaspoon dried rosemary
- Salt and pepper to taste
- Dysphagia-friendly sides such as mashed potatoes or soft vegetables (optional)

Instructions:

- Get the chicken ready: Add the skinless, boneless chicken thighs or breasts to the slow cooker.
- Incorporate Aromatics: Divide the minced garlic and finely chopped onions among the chicken pieces in the slow cooker.
- Add the broth: To keep the chicken moist while it cooks slowly, cover it with low-sodium chicken broth.
- The season: For a tasty and fragrant seasoning, add salt, pepper, dried thyme, and dried rosemary to the chicken.
- Cook Slowly: After putting the slow cooker on low heat for 6 to 8 hours, or until the chicken is fork-tender, shred it easily.
- Shred the chicken: After the chicken is cooked, shred it right in the slow cooker using two forks. The chicken should be so delicate that it falls apart easily after a long time.

- Modify the seasoning: After tasting the shredded chicken, taste again and adjust the seasoning with more salt or pepper to taste.
- Serve: Serve the Slow-Cooked Shredded Chicken by itself or with sides such as soft vegetables or mashed potatoes that are suitable for those with dysphagia.
- Savor the Sensual Joy: Savor the rich flavors that can only be achieved through slow cooking as you sink your teeth into the succulent delicacy of Slow-Cooked Shredded Chicken.

Baked Salmon with Lemon Dill Sauce

Ingredients:

For Baked Salmon:

- 4 salmon fillets, skinless
- 2 tablespoons olive oil
- Salt and pepper to taste

- 1 lemon, thinly sliced
- Fresh dill for garnish

For Lemon Dill Sauce:

- 1/2 cup Greek yogurt or a non-dairy
  alternative
- 1 tablespoon fresh dill, finely
  chopped
- 1 tablespoon lemon juice
- 1 teaspoon Dijon mustard
- Salt and pepper to taste

Instructions:

For Baked Salmon:

- Warm up the oven:Turn the oven on
  to 375°F, or 190°C.
- Get the salmon ready:Using a paper
  towel, pat the salmon fillets dry.
  Transfer them to a parchment
  paper-lined baking sheet.
- Olive oil drizzled on top:Make sure
  the salmon fillets are thoroughly

coated by drizzling them with olive oil. To taste, add salt and pepper for seasoning.

- Add slices of lemon to the layer:Top each salmon fillet with a tiny slice of lemon to give it a citrus flavor burst while it bakes.
- Cook:Bake for 15 to 20 minutes, or until the salmon is cooked through and flake readily with a fork, in an oven that has been warmed.
- Accessory:For a burst of herbal freshness, sprinkle some fresh dill over the cooked salmon.
- Regarding Lemon Dill Sauce:Get the sauce ready:Greek yogurt or a non dairy substitute, fresh dill cut finely, lemon juice, Dijon mustard, salt, and pepper should all be combined in a small bowl.
- Blend Well:Mix the ingredients until a smooth, well-blended sauce is achieved.

- To Assist:Salmon on a plate:Transfer the cooked salmon fillets to platters for serving.
- Pour Sauce Over:For a tasty and creamy side dish, drizzle each salmon fillet with the Lemon Dill Sauce.
- Optional garnish:Garnish with extra fresh dill, if desired, for an extra whiff of herbaceous flavor.
- Present and Savor:Savor the harmonic blend of soft salmon and the zesty, vibrant flavors of the sauce as you indulge in the culinary adventure that is Baked Salmon with Lemon Dill Sauce.

Turkey and Sweet Potato Mash

Ingredients:

- 1 pound ground turkey
- 2 cups sweet potatoes, peeled and diced

- 1/2 cup low-sodium chicken broth
- 1 tablespoon olive oil
- 1 onion, finely chopped
- 2 cloves garlic, minced
- 1 teaspoon dried thyme
- Salt and pepper to taste
- Chopped fresh parsley for garnish (optional)

Instructions:

- Get the sweet potatoes ready:Sweet potatoes should be peeled and chopped into uniformly small pieces.
- Prepare Sweet Potatoes:Cook the sweet potatoes in a pot of boiling water until they are soft. After draining, set away.
- Sauté garlic and onions:Heat the olive oil in a big skillet over medium heat. Add the minced garlic and finely chopped onions, and sauté until aromatic and transparent.

- Cook Turkey Ground:Using a spoon, crumble the turkey ground and add it to the skillet. Cook the turkey until it is thoroughly done and browned.
- The season: To add savory flavors to the turkey mixture, sprinkle it with salt, pepper, and dried thyme.
- Sweet potatoes mashed:To make the cooked sweet potatoes smooth and creamy, mash them and add low-sodium chicken broth.
- Mix sweet potatoes and turkey together:To create a pleasing fusion of flavors and textures, mix the mashed sweet potatoes with the seasoned ground turkey.
- Modify the seasoning:After giving the mixture a taste, adjust the seasoning by adding additional salt or pepper to your taste.
- Optional garnish:For an optional pop of color and extra freshness, sprinkle chopped fresh parsley over the Turkey and Sweet Potato Mash.

- Present and Savor:Serve the Turkey and Sweet Potato Mash and enjoy the comforting contrast of the creamy sweet potatoes and the robust turkey.

Lentil and Vegetable Stew

Ingredients:

- 1 cup dried green or brown lentils, rinsed
- 4 cups low-sodium vegetable broth
- 2 carrots, peeled and diced
- 2 celery stalks, diced
- 1 onion, finely chopped
- 2 cloves garlic, minced
- 1 cup diced tomatoes (fresh or canned)
- 1 cup sweet potatoes, peeled and diced
- 1 teaspoon ground cumin
- 1 teaspoon smoked paprika
- 1 bay leaf

- Salt and pepper to taste
- 2 tablespoons olive oil
- Fresh parsley for garnish (optional)

Instructions:

- Get the lentils ready:After rinsing with cold water, set aside the dry lentils.
- Aromatics in sauté:Warm up the olive oil in a big pot over medium heat. Add the minced garlic and finely chopped onions, and sauté until aromatic and transparent.
- Include Veggies:Add the chopped celery, carrots, and sweet potatoes to the pot. Cook until the vegetables begin to soften, about 5 to 7 minutes.
- The season:Add a little bit of salt, pepper, smoked paprika, and ground cumin to the vegetables to give them a flavorful, smokey taste.
- Add the broth and lentils:To the pot, add the chopped tomatoes, low-sodium vegetable broth, bay

leaf, and rinsed lentils. Mix thoroughly to blend.

- Reduce: After bringing the mixture to a boil, lower the heat so that it simmers. When the lentils and veggies are soft, cover the saucepan and simmer for 25 to 30 minutes.
- Modify the seasoning:After tasting the stew, taste again and adjust the seasoning by adding additional salt or pepper to suit your taste.
- Present and Garnish:Spoon the Vegetable and Lentil Stew into individual bowls. Add some fresh parsley as a garnish if you want to add some color and freshness.
- Savor the Wholesome Joy:Savor the nutritious blend of lentils, veggies, and flavorful spices as you sink your teeth into the heartiness of Lentil and Vegetable Stew.

This adaption is great for those with dysphagia and adds a pleasant variety of flavors and textures. The variety of vegetables brings color and minerals, while the lentils give a basis that's high in protein. Lentil and Vegetable Stew exemplifies the idea of "Savoring Soft Delights," providing both culinary satisfaction and ease of ingestion for seniors with specific dietary requirements. It can be eaten as a comfortable meal on its own or as part of a larger dining experience.

CHAPTER 4

DELICATE SIDE DISHES

Mashed Cauliflower with Garlic Butter

Ingredients:

- 1 large head of cauliflower, cut into florets
- 2 cloves garlic, minced
- 2 tablespoons unsalted butter or olive oil
- 1/4 cup low-sodium chicken or vegetable broth
- Salt and pepper to taste
- Chopped chives or parsley for garnish (optional)

Instructions:

- Cooked cauliflower in steam:When the cauliflower florets are fork-tender, steam them. You may microwave this with a tiny quantity of water or use a steamer basket over boiling water.

- Crush the cauliflower:After steaming, transfer the cauliflower to a big basin. To get the correct consistency, mash the cauliflower using an immersion blender or a potato masher.
- Get the garlic butter ready:Heat a small saucepan over low heat to melt unsalted butter. Add the minced garlic and cook, stirring, for one to two minutes, or until fragrant.
- Mix the ingredients together:Cover the mashed cauliflower with the garlic butter mixture. Stirring constantly, add low-sodium chicken or vegetable broth until the mixture has a smooth, creamy consistency.
- The season:To taste, add salt and pepper to the mashed cauliflower.

Tailor the seasoning to your personal taste.

- Optional garnish:Garnish the Mashed Cauliflower with Garlic Butter with chopped parsley or chives if you want to add some more freshness and color.
- Present and Savor:Ladle the Mashed Cauliflower with Garlic Butter onto plates and enjoy the flavorful union of the garlic butter and the creamy cauliflower.

Creamed Spinach

Ingredients:
- 1 pound fresh spinach, washed and stems removed
- 2 tablespoons unsalted butter
- 2 tablespoons all-purpose flour
- 1 cup whole milk or a non-dairy alternative
- 1/4 cup grated Parmesan cheese
- 1/4 teaspoon ground nutmeg

- Salt and pepper to taste
- Optional: Dash of ground cayenne pepper for a subtle heat

Instructions:

- Blanch the spinach:Blanch fresh spinach in a pot of boiling water for one to two minutes, or until wilted. To stop the heating process, quickly move the spinach to a bowl of icy water. After blanching the spinach, drain and chop.
- Get the cream sauce ready: Unsalted butter should be melted in a saucepan over medium heat. Add all-purpose flour and mix to make a roux, stirring constantly. The roux should be cooked for one to two minutes, or until it turns pale golden.
- Include Milk:Stir add whole milk or a dairy-free substitute for the roux gradually, making sure to mix it in smoothly. Whisk the mixture continuously until it thickens.

- Add nutmeg and Parmesan cheeses:To the cream sauce, add ground nutmeg and grated Parmesan cheese. Mix until the cheese has melted and the mixture has a hint of warmth from the nutmeg.
- Mix with spinach:Make sure the spinach is evenly coated with the delicious mixture by folding the chopped, blanched spinach into the cream sauce.
- The season: To taste, add more salt and pepper to the creamed spinach. If preferred, add a small amount of ground cayenne pepper for a sense of gentle spice.
- Cook and Present:To allow the flavors to mingle, boil the creamed spinach for a few minutes. Spoon the creamy spinach into serving bowls or onto plates after it's heated thoroughly.
- Optional garnish: For an additional flavor boost, feel free to add a dash

of nutmeg or an extra sprinkling of Parmesan cheese.

- Present and Savor:Enjoy Creamed Spinach's velvety smoothness and delicious depth, relishing every morsel of this dysphagia-friendly dish.

Soft Quinoa Pilaf

Ingredients:

- 1 cup quinoa, rinsed
- 2 cups low-sodium chicken or vegetable broth
- 1 tablespoon olive oil
- 1 small onion, finely chopped
- 2 cloves garlic, minced
- 1 carrot, peeled and finely diced
- 1 zucchini, finely diced
- 1/2 cup cooked and finely shredded chicken (optional)
- 1/4 cup chopped fresh parsley
- Salt and pepper to taste

Instructions:

- Wash Quinoa:In order to get rid of any bitterness, rinse the quinoa in cold water.
- Prepare Quinoa:Quinoa and low-sodium chicken or veggie broth should be combined in a saucepan. After bringing to a boil, lower the heat, cover, and simmer the quinoa for 15 to 20 minutes, or until it is tender and the liquid has been absorbed. Using a fork, fluff.
- Aromatics in sauté:Heat the olive oil in a separate pan over medium heat. Add the minced garlic and finely diced onions, and sauté until aromatic and translucent.
- Include Veggies:Add the zucchini and carrots, chopped fine, to the pan. Cook until the vegetables are tender, about 5 to 7 minutes.
- Mix Quinoa with the Veggies:Mix the cooked quinoa and the sautéed vegetables together to form a

cohesive blend. Add cooked and finely shredded chicken if you want to increase the protein content.

- The season:To ensure that the flavor profile of the Soft Quinoa Pilaf is well-balanced, season with salt and pepper to taste.
- Add parsley as a garnish:Add chopped fresh parsley to the pilaf to give it a vibrant splash of color and freshness.
- Cook and Present:To allow the flavors to mingle, cook the Soft Quinoa Pilaf for a few minutes. Spoon the pilaf into serving bowls or onto plates once it's heated thoroughly.
- Present and Savor:Savor the nutritious combination of quinoa and a variety of veggies as you indulge in the soft and filling goodness of Soft Quinoa Pilaf.

Roasted Beets with Orange Glaze

Ingredients:

- 4 medium-sized beets, peeled and cut into wedges
- 2 tablespoons olive oil
- Salt and pepper to taste
- Zest of one orange
- 1/3 cup freshly squeezed orange juice
- 2 tablespoons honey or maple syrup
- 1 tablespoon balsamic vinegar
- Chopped fresh parsley for garnish (optional)

Instructions:

- Warm up the oven:Set oven temperature to 400°F, or 200°C.
- Get the beets ready:Making sure the beets are all the same size for even roasting, peel and cut them into wedges.

- Beets roasted:Put the wedges of beetroot onto a baking sheet. Add a drizzle of olive oil and season with pepper and salt. Toss to evenly coat the beets. Bake the beets for 25 to 30 minutes in a preheated oven, or until they are soft and have a hint of caramelization.
- Get the orange glaze ready:Orange zest, freshly squeezed orange juice, honey (or maple syrup), and balsamic vinegar should all be combined in a small pot. Over medium heat, bring the mixture to a simmer, stirring from time to time. Simmer for five to seven minutes, or until the glazing somewhat thickens.
- Dredge beets in glaze:After roasting, move the beets to a serving bowl. Drizzle the roasted beets with the orange glaze and toss gently to coat the beets with the delicious glaze.
- Optional garnish:For an optional pop of color and extra freshness, sprinkle

chopped fresh parsley on top of the Roasted Beets with Orange Glaze.

- Present and Savor:Present the Roasted Beets with Orange Glaze and enjoy the well-balanced taste of earthy, sweet beets and zesty orange glaze.

This adaptation is dysphagia-friendly and offers a delicious blend of textures and flavors. The orange glaze's zesty richness accentuates the delicate, caramelized roasted beets. Roasted Beets with Orange Glaze is the epitome of "Savoring Soft Delights," as it can be enjoyed both as an easy-to-eat side dish or as part of a well-planned meal that accommodates seniors with special dietary needs.

CHAPTER 5

COMFORTING MAIN COURSES

Soft Meatballs in Tomato Sauce

Ingredients:

For Meatballs:

- 1 pound ground beef or ground turkey
- 1/2 cup breadcrumbs (ensure they are finely ground for a softer texture)
- 1/4 cup grated Parmesan cheese
- 1/4 cup milk or a non-dairy alternative
- 1 large egg
- 2 tablespoons finely chopped fresh parsley
- 1 clove garlic, minced
- Salt and pepper to taste

For Tomato Sauce:

- 2 cups tomato sauce (homemade or store-bought)
- 1 tablespoon olive oil
- 1 small onion, finely chopped
- 2 cloves garlic, minced
- 1 teaspoon dried oregano
- Salt and pepper to taste
- Fresh basil for garnish (optional)

Instructions:

For Meatballs:

- Warm up the oven: Turn the oven on to 375°F, or 190°C.
- Get the meatball mixture ready. Ground beef or turkey, breadcrumbs, grated Parmesan cheese, milk, egg, minced garlic, chopped fresh parsley, salt, and pepper should all be combined in a big bowl. Blend until thoroughly blended.

- Form Meatballs:Make sure the meatballs are uniformly proportioned for even cooking by shaping them into tiny, bite-sized balls.
- Cook Meatballs in the Oven:Arrange the meatballs onto a parchment paper-lined baking sheet. Bake for 15 to 20 minutes, or until the meatballs are tender and thoroughly cooked, in a preheated oven.
- Regarding Tomato Sauce:Aromatics in sauté:Olive oil should be heated in a saucepan over medium heat. Add the minced garlic and finely diced onions, and sauté until aromatic and translucent.
- Include tomato sauce:Stirring to blend with the sautéed aromatics, pour the tomato sauce into the pot.
- The season: Add salt, pepper, and dried oregano to the tomato sauce for seasoning. Tailor the seasoning to your personal taste.

- Reduce:Simmer the tomato sauce for ten to fifteen minutes so that the flavors can combine and the sauce becomes a little thicker.
- To Assist:Mix sauce and meatballs together:Make sure the baked meatballs are equally coated by gently dipping them into the tomato sauce.
- Together, Simmer:Give the meatballs ten more minutes to boil in the tomato sauce so they can absorb the flavor.
- Optional garnish:For a pop of herbal flavor, feel free to top the Soft Meatballs in Tomato Sauce with some fresh basil.
- Present and Savor:Savor the tender sweetness of the meatballs in the rich tomato sauce by serving the Soft Meatballs in Tomato Sauce over mashed potatoes or soft noodles.

Tender Beef Stew with Root Vegetables

Ingredients:

- 1.5 pounds stewing beef, cut into bite-sized cubes
- 2 tablespoons vegetable oil
- 1 onion, finely chopped
- 2 cloves garlic, minced
- 4 cups beef broth (low-sodium)
- 1 cup carrots, peeled and diced
- 1 cup potatoes, peeled and diced
- 1 cup parsnips, peeled and diced
- 1 cup turnips, peeled and diced
- 1 teaspoon dried thyme
- 1 bay leaf
- Salt and pepper to taste
- Chopped fresh parsley for garnish (optional)

Instructions:

- Seared beef:Vegetable oil should be heated over medium-high heat in a big pot. Sear the meat cubes until they are browned all over. This gives the stew more flavor.
- Aromatics in sauté:Add minced garlic and finely diced onions to the saucepan. The onions should be transparent and fragrant after sautéing.
- Include Beef Broth:Add the beef broth and scrape up any tasty pieces from the bottom of the kettle to deglaze it.
- Add Some Vegetables:Add diced turnips, parsnips, potatoes, and carrots to the pot. Mix the beef and broth together by stirring.
- The season:Add the bay leaf, a pinch of dried thyme, and salt & pepper to taste when preparing the stew. To ensure the flavors merge, stir thoroughly.

- Reduce:After bringing the stew to a boil, turn down the heat. Once the vegetables and meat are soft and the beef is cooked, cover the pot and simmer for one and a half to two hours.
- Modify the seasoning:After tasting the stew, taste again and adjust the seasoning with extra salt or pepper to taste.
- Optional garnish:For a pop of color and more freshness, you can optionally add chopped fresh parsley to the Tender Beef Stew with Root Vegetables.
- Present and Savor:Pour the stew into bowls and enjoy the fragrant broth, the combination of root vegetables and the tender beef.

Chicken and Rice Casserole

Ingredients:

- 1.5 pounds boneless, skinless chicken breasts, cut into bite-sized pieces
- 1 cup white rice, uncooked
- 2 cups low-sodium chicken broth
- 1 cup carrots, peeled and finely diced
- 1 cup peas (fresh or frozen)
- 1/2 cup celery, finely chopped
- 1/2 cup unsalted butter
- 1/2 cup all-purpose flour
- 2 cups whole milk or a non-dairy alternative
- 1 teaspoon garlic powder
- Salt and pepper to taste
- Chopped fresh parsley for garnish (optional)

Instructions:

- Warm up the oven:Set the oven's temperature to 175°C/350°F.
- Cook the chicken:Cook the bite-sized chicken pieces in a skillet over

medium heat until the chicken is no longer pink in the middle. Put aside.

- Get the rice ready:Cook the white rice in a different pot as directed on the package, using low-sodium chicken broth for water to give it more taste.
- Steam-cooked veggies:Dice the carrots and peas finely and steam until soft. Put aside.
- Create a Creamy Sauce:Melt the unsalted butter in a skillet over a medium heat. To make a roux, add the all-purpose flour and mix. Stir in whole milk or a non dairy substitute gradually to achieve a creamy and smooth texture. To taste, add pepper, salt, and garlic powder.
- Mix the ingredients together:Steamed carrots and peas, cooked rice, diced celery, and cooked chicken should all be combined in a big mixing dish. After adding the creamy sauce to the

mixture, carefully fold everything together until it is well coated.

- Move to a Casserole Plate:Spread the mixture equally in a casserole dish that has been buttered.
- Cook:Bake for 30 to 35 minutes, or until the top of the dish is golden brown and bubbling, in a preheated oven.
- Optional garnish:You can optionally add some chopped fresh parsley to the Chicken and Rice Casserole to give it some color and flavor.
- Present and Savor:Ladle the dish onto plates and enjoy every cozy taste of the fluffy rice, creamy deliciousness, and soft chicken.

Eggplant Parmesan Puree

Ingredients:

- 1 large eggplant, peeled and diced
- 2 tablespoons olive oil

- 2 cloves garlic, minced
- 1 cup tomato sauce (homemade or store-bought)
- 1/2 cup grated Parmesan cheese
- 1/2 cup mozzarella cheese, shredded
- 1 teaspoon dried oregano
- Salt and pepper to taste
- Fresh basil for garnish (optional)

Instructions:

- Warm up the oven:Set oven temperature to 400°F, or 200°C.
- Grilled eggplant:Arrange the chopped eggplant onto a baking tray. Sprinkle with salt and pepper, drizzle with olive oil, and toss to coat evenly. Roast the eggplant for 20 to 25 minutes, or until it's soft and beginning to turn brown, in a preheated oven.
- Sauté the garlic:Heat a tiny bit of olive oil in a skillet over medium

heat. When aromatic, add the minced garlic and sauté it.

- Mix the ingredients together:To the skillet with the sautéed garlic, add the roasted eggplant. Add the dried oregano, shredded mozzarella, grated Parmesan cheese, and tomato sauce. Mixing the components thoroughly requires stirring.
- Reduce:Simmer the mixture for 5 to 7 minutes to allow the cheeses to melt and the flavors to combine.
- Mix to a Puree:Puree the mixture until it's smooth by transferring it to a blender or using an immersion blender. To acquire the right consistency, feel free to add a tiny bit of vegetable or chicken broth.
- Modify the seasoning:After tasting the eggplant parmesan puree, taste it again and adjust the seasoning by adding additional salt or pepper to taste.

- Optional garnish:To add a hint of herbal freshness, you can optionally garnish the puree with fresh basil.
- Present and Savor:Pour the Eggplant Parmesan Puree into bowls and enjoy the rich, flavorful sauce with a smooth consistency that is reminiscent of a traditional dish.

This pureed version offers a delicious blend of Italian tastes that is suitable for those with dysphagia. The puree of roasted eggplant, tomato sauce, and cheese is filling and nutritious. Eggplant Parmesan Puree captures the spirit of "Savoring Soft Delights," making it ideal for seniors with special dietary needs and a delicious meal to eat on its own or as part of a well-planned dining experience.

CHAPTER 6

DELECTABLE DESSERTS

Poached Pears in Vanilla Sauce

Ingredients:

- 4 ripe but firm pears, peeled and halved
- 1 cup water
- 1 cup apple juice
- 1/2 cup granulated sugar
- 1 vanilla bean, split lengthwise (or 1 teaspoon vanilla extract)
- Zest of one lemon
- 1 tablespoon cornstarch (optional, for thickening)
- Whipped cream or vanilla yogurt for serving (optional)
- Chopped nuts or mint for garnish (optional)

Instructions:

- Get the pears ready:After removing the seeds and core, peel and cut the pears in half. Make sure the pears are firm but not overripe.
- Stealing Liquid:Place water, apple juice, granulated sugar, split vanilla bean (or vanilla extract), and zest of lemon in a pot. Over medium heat, bring the mixture to a moderate simmer.
- Pick Your Own Pears:Put the pear halves into the poaching liquid with care. Simmer the pears for 15 to 20 minutes, or until they are soft but not mushy. For even poaching, rotate the pears from time to time.
- Take the pears out:After poaching, use a slotted spoon to remove the pears from the liquor and set them aside.
- Sauce à la vanille:Take the vanilla bean out of the poaching liquor if you're using one. Make a slurry out of

cornstarch and a tiny bit of water if you want the sauce to be thicker. After adding the slurry to the poaching liquid, boil it until it thickens a little.

- Serve:Place the halves of poached pears on serving dishes. Over the pears, drizzle the vanilla sauce.
- Optional garnish:Garnish with a dollop of vanilla yogurt or whipped cream, if desired. For an additional elegant and flavorful touch, add a sprig of mint or sprinkle chopped nuts on top.
- Present and Savor:Present the Poached Pears in Vanilla Sauce, relishing the subtle sweetness of the pears and the fragrant depth of the sauce enhanced with vanilla.

Silken Chocolate Pudding

Ingredients:
- 1/2 cup granulated sugar

- 1/4 cup unsweetened cocoa powder
- 3 tablespoons cornstarch
- 1/8 teaspoon salt
- 2 cups whole milk or a non-dairy alternative
- 1/2 cup dark chocolate, finely chopped
- 1 teaspoon vanilla extract
- Whipped cream or a dollop of yogurt for serving (optional)
- Chocolate shavings or berries for garnish (optional)

Instructions:

- Mix the dry ingredients together:Granulated sugar, unsweetened cocoa powder, cornstarch, and salt should all be thoroughly mixed in a basin.
- Warm Milk:The entire milk should be heated in a saucepan over medium heat until it barely starts to simmer. Keep it from boiling.
- Add the Dry Ingredients:Making sure there are no lumps, gradually whisk

the dry ingredient combination into the simmering milk.

- Prepare the Pudding Base:Stirring continually, simmer the mixture over medium heat until it thickens. This could take five to seven minutes.
- Add some chocolate:After turning off the heat, transfer the coarsely chopped dark chocolate to the pudding base in the saucepan. Mix the mixture until it becomes smooth and the chocolate has melted.
- Include vanilla extract:Add the vanilla extract and stir to give the pudding a lovely scent.
- Stress (Optional):You can strain the pudding through a fine-mesh sieve to get rid of any possible lumps for an extra smooth texture.
- Divide into Cups:Transfer the smooth chocolate pudding into separate serving basins or cups.
- Relax:To stop a skin from forming, cover the cups with plastic wrap,

making sure it contacts the pudding's surface. Refrigerate for a minimum of two hours or until solidified.

- Serve:You can choose to add a dollop of yogurt or whipped cream on top of the Silken Chocolate Pudding. For an added touch of elegance, garnish with fresh berries or chocolate shavings.
- Present and Savor:Savor every spoonful of Silken Chocolate Pudding's rich chocolate taste and silky texture as you enjoy this delectable delicacy.

Berry Smoothie Sorbet

Ingredients:

- 2 cups mixed berries (strawberries, blueberries, raspberries)
- 1/4 cup honey or maple syrup

- 1 cup vanilla yogurt (non-dairy alternatives can be used)
- 1 tablespoon fresh lemon juice
- Fresh mint leaves for garnish (optional)

Instructions:

- Get the berries ready:If used, wash and shell the strawberries. In a blender, combine the mixed berries.
- Mix berries:Puree the berries in a blender until they form a bright berry puree.
- Put in some sweetener:Pour maple syrup or honey over the berry puree. To include the sweetener, blend once more.
- Add Yogurt:Mix the berry combination with the vanilla yogurt. Blend the mixture until it's well incorporated and smooth.
- Incorporate Lemon Juice:Add freshly squeezed lemon juice to the mixer. Lemon juice gives the sorbet a zesty,

refreshing twist, so blend just long enough to incorporate it.

- Taste and Modify:If necessary, taste the sorbet mixture and add more honey, maple syrup, or lemon juice to modify the sweetness or sharpness.
- Freeze:Transfer the sorbet mixture of the berry smoothie into a shallow dish that may be frozen. Using a spatula, level the surface.
- Freeze till determined:The sorbet should harden up after at least four to six hours of setting time in the freezer.
- Serve:Allow the sorbet to soften slightly at room temperature for a few minutes before serving. Pour Berry Smoothie Sorbet into glasses or bowls using a spoon.
- Optional garnish:For an extra burst of herbal freshness, feel free to garnish with fresh mint leaves.
- Present and Savor:Savor the natural sweetness of mixed berries with each

scoop of Berry Smoothie Sorbet's cool, refreshing flavor.

Cinnamon Applesauce Delight

Ingredients:

- 4 medium-sized apples, peeled, cored, and diced
- 1/4 cup water
- 2 tablespoons lemon juice
- 2 tablespoons honey or maple syrup
- 1 teaspoon ground cinnamon
- 1/4 teaspoon vanilla extract (optional)
- Pinch of salt

Instructions:

- Get the apples ready:Cut the apples into uniformly sized pieces after peeling and cored.
- Simmering Apples: Diced apples, water, lemon juice, honey or maple syrup, ground cinnamon, vanilla extract (if using), and a dash of salt

should all be combined in a
saucepan.

- Cook until the meat is tender.Over
medium heat, bring the mixture to a
moderate simmer. Once the apples
are soft and easily mashed, cover the
saucepan and cook for 15 to 20
minutes.
- Dicing Apples:When the apples are
soft, mash them to the consistency
you want with a fork or potato
masher. You can use an immersion
blender to achieve a smoother
texture.
- Modify the cinnamon and
sweetness:If necessary, taste the
applesauce and add extra honey or
maple syrup to adjust the sweetness.
Similarly, taste and adjust the
cinnamon.
- Optional: Simmer to Thicken:You can
boil the applesauce uncovered for a
few more minutes to thicken it if it's
too runny.

- Nice:When the cinnamon applesauce delight reaches room temperature, let it cool.
- Keep cold:Before serving, let the applesauce sit in the fridge for at least one hour. Applesauce that has been chilled will taste better.
- Serve:Pour the Applesauce Delight with cinnamon into bowls or cups.
- Optional garnish:Garnish with a small pinch of extra cinnamon, if desired.
- Present and Savor:Savor the natural sweetness and fragrant cinnamon notes of cinnamon as you indulge in the warm and comforting flavor of cinnamon applesauce.

CHAPTER 7

HYDRATION AND NOURISHMENT

- Hydration: Liquids with thickening, Assist medical practitioners in determining the appropriate liquid thickness level. Liquids that have thickened can be simpler to swallow, which lowers the chance of aspiration.

- Taking Regular Drinks of Water:Urge people to drink water in small amounts throughout the day. Staying hydrated is important for general health and can facilitate swallowing.

- Hydration Timetable:Create a water-drinking regimen. Maintaining a regular schedule aids in preventing dehydration, which exacerbates swallowing difficulties.

- Infusions of Flavor:Add natural flavors like lemon, cucumber, or mint to water to make it more enticing. This may enhance the pleasure of maintaining hydration.

- Adjustable Cups:Use straws or cups that are adapted for people who have trouble swallowing. By regulating the flow of liquids, these tools help make drinking easier to handle.

Food:

- Diet Modified by Texture:Work together with medical experts to develop a food that has been changed in texture according to each person's ability to swallow. Textures like soft, pureed, or minced may be involved.
- Rich in Nutrients Foods:Make nutrient-dense meals a priority to make sure your diet includes the necessary vitamins and minerals. Soft fruits, veggies, and foods high in protein are great selections.
- Blended or pureed options:Add items that have been blended or pureed to your diet. Smoothies, soups, and pureed veggies can offer a range of

flavors in a form that is simple to consume.

- Little, Regular Meals:Choose to eat smaller meals more often during the day. By cutting back on the quantity of food eaten at each sitting, this method can help with swallowing.
- Avert Hard or Dry Foods:Avoid foods that are firm or dry as they can cause choking. Choose foods that are soft, moist, and simpler to chew and swallow.
- Track Your Weight:Pay special attention to your weight and nutritional state. When there are worries about undernourishment or weight loss, work with medical practitioners to modify the diet.
- Supplements for nutrition:If you need more calories and nutrients, think about taking nutritional supplements or drinking smoothies. Make sure these supplements follow the recommended dietary guidelines.

- Speech Pathology:Enroll in speech therapy courses that address managing dysphagia. Speech therapists can offer exercises and methods to enhance the ability to swallow.

General Advice
- Speak with Medical Experts:To create and adjust food plans according to specific needs, consult medical specialists such as speech therapists and nutritionists.
- Dining Area:Establish a serene and cozy dining area. Reduce outside distractions to help you concentrate on the food and encourage healthy, pleasurable eating.
- Engagement of Family and Caregivers:Incorporate caregivers and family members into the dysphagia control strategy. Inform them about dietary limitations, suggested foods, and techniques for staying hydrated.

CONCLUSION

When we turn to the last page of "Savoring Soft Delights: Nourishing Recipes for Seniors with Dysphagia," we take stock of the culinary adventure designed specifically for those who struggle with swallowing. This cookbook is a tribute to the idea that every meal should be a source of happiness, solace, and nourishment regardless of dietary restrictions rather than just a compilation of recipes.

Mealtimes can become a source of monotony and frustration for seniors who are managing their dysphagia. Our goal in writing these pages has been to change that experience. Every recipe is a meticulously composed symphony of tastes, textures, and nutrients that are meant to fulfill dietary needs but also make dining a pleasurable and fulfilling ritual.

Our dedication to offering options that are both palatable and simple to swallow has guided us as we've progressed through the chapters, from soups that warm the spirit to sweets that sweeten life's moments. It's a tribute to the pleasure of indulging in delicate treats, where each mouthful embodies the spirit of careful planning and the wish to make every dinner an occasion for delight.

We would like to express our appreciation to the elders, caregivers, and medical professionals that helped and motivated us with this initiative. This culinary initiative has been motivated by your experiences, insights, and commitment to improving the lives of people with dysphagia.

We hope you will continue experimenting with these recipes as we complete this chapter, customizing them to your own tastes and extending your repertoire of delicious dysphagia-friendly dishes. May every meal serve as a celebration of life, an occasion to relish, and a reminder that everyone may still enjoy delicious food despite dietary restrictions.

I hope that "Savoring Soft Delights" serves as a source of inspiration, offering not just recipes but also a road map to a future in which each bite is satisfying and fulfilling. Cheers to the elderly and their ongoing quest to appreciate life's little pleasures.

www.ingramcontent.com/pod-product-compliance
Lightning Source LLC
Chambersburg PA
CBHW061002260726
48661CB00005B/1998